Even-Heat

The Key to Perfectly Cooked Dishes

M.A. Gorre

Contents

Chapter One

Introduction

Cooking is an intricate blend of artistry and science, where flavors harmonize, textures entice, and aromas tantalize the senses. At the core of this culinary symphony lies the essential ingredient that can make or break your dishes: heat. Imagine a chef's kitchen as a grand orchestra, with various instruments representing different cooking methods and appliances. Just as a maestro needs precise control over each instrument to create beautiful music, a skilled chef requires mastery over the element of heat to craft perfect dishes.

This book embarks on a culinary journey, delving deep into the heart of cooking, into the very essence of culinary excellence—achieving even heat. Over the following pages, we will explore the science behind heat, unveil its transformative powers, and teach you how to harness it with finesse, resulting in dishes that are consistently and flawlessly cooked.

The journey begins by unraveling the science of heat, from the basics of heat transfer to the role of temperature in culinary alchemy. With a solid understanding of these principles, we will dive into the practical aspects of achieving even heat in your kitchen. From choosing the right cookware to mastering essential cooking techniques, you'll build a strong foundation.

Next, we'll explore various cooking environments, from stovetops to ovens, grills, and specialty appliances. You'll gain insights into how to achieve even heat on different platforms, whether it's coaxing the perfect flame on your stovetop, roasting to perfection in your oven, or infusing smoky flavor on your grill.

Common cooking challenges often test our culinary skills. We'll equip you with the knowledge and techniques to overcome these obstacles, ensuring your dishes consistently turn out delicious. Perfecting your timing is another crucial aspect of cooking, and we'll share tips and tricks for mastering this art.

To put theory into practice, we've included a collection of recipes that highlight the power of even heat. From breakfast classics to delectable desserts, each recipe is carefully crafted to help you refine your even heating skills. Step-by-step instructions and cooking tips ensure that your culinary creations are nothing short of perfection.

Lastly, we'll explore the broader applications of even heat beyond the kitchen. Whether you're interested in DIY projects, home brewing, or simply conducting fascinating heat-related experiments, the principles you've learned here will prove invaluable.

In conclusion, "Even Heat: The Key to Perfectly Cooked Dishes" is your comprehensive guide to understanding and mastering the fundamental element of cooking. Beyond being a cookbook, this book is a journey of culinary discovery, an exploration of the science and artistry of cooking. With the knowledge and skills you'll acquire, you'll be well-equipped to achieve culinary excellence in your own kitchen. So, let's embark on this culinary adventure together and unlock the secrets of even heat.

Chapter Two

Why Even Heat Matters in Cooking

Even heat is a foundational and crucial aspect of cooking for several reasons. Understanding why even heat matters in cooking is essential for anyone looking to prepare delicious and consistent meals. Here are some key reasons:

1. **Uniform Cooking:** Even heat ensures that all parts of a dish receive consistent and uniform cooking. This means that every bite of your meal will have the same level of doneness and flavor, eliminating the risk of overcooked or undercooked portions.

2. **Precise Control:** Cooking is often about precise control of temperature. Even heat allows you to maintain a steady temperature throughout the cooking process, giving you control over how ingredients transform. This is particularly impor-

tant for techniques like sautéing, simmering, and braising.

3. **Flavor Development:** Many dishes rely on the gradual development of flavors through cooking. Even heat helps ingredients release their flavors evenly, resulting in a well-balanced and harmonious taste. For example, caramelization of sugars in onions or the Maillard reaction in meat both require even heat for optimal flavor.

4. **Texture Consistency:** Even heat contributes to consistent texture in dishes. Whether you're searing a steak to achieve a crispy crust while keeping the inside tender or baking a cake to perfection, even heat ensures that textures are uniform.

5. **Efficient Cooking:** Even heat leads to efficient cooking. When heat is distributed evenly, you can reduce cooking times, saving energy and making meal preparation more efficient.

6. **Avoiding Hot Spots and Cold Spots:** Uneven heat can result in hot spots and cold spots within your cookware or oven. This can lead to unpredictable cooking outcomes, with some parts of the dish cooking faster than others. Even heat minimizes these discrepancies.

7. **Preventing Food Waste:** Cooking with even heat helps prevent food waste. When food is evenly cooked, there's less chance of burning or overcooking, which can make ingredients unpalatable and lead to waste.

8. **Consistency in Recipes:** When you're following a recipe, achieving even heat ensures that your results match the in-

tended outcome described in the recipe. This consistency is especially important for those who enjoy cooking as a hobby or for special occasions.

9. **Professional Results at Home:** Even heat is a hallmark of professional cooking. By mastering even heat in your home kitchen, you can replicate the quality and consistency found in restaurant-quality dishes.

10. **Versatility:** Whether you're roasting vegetables, searing meats, baking pastries, or simmering sauces, even heat is a versatile requirement. It's essential across a wide range of cooking techniques and cuisines.

In summary, even heat matters in cooking because it directly impacts the taste, texture, and consistency of your dishes. It allows you to have precise control over the cooking process, resulting in better-cooked meals and more successful culinary endeavors. Whether you're a novice or an experienced cook, understanding and achieving even heat is a fundamental skill that can elevate your cooking to a higher level.

Chapter Three

How This Book Can Help You Master Even Heat?

This book, "Even Heat: The Key to Perfectly Cooked Dishes," is designed to be your comprehensive guide to mastering even heat in cooking. It provides you with the knowledge, techniques, and practical tips needed to achieve consistent and delicious results in your culinary endeavors. Here's how this book can help you master even heat:

1. **Understanding the Science**: This book starts by explaining the science behind heat and heat transfer. You'll gain a deep understanding of how heat moves through different materials and how temperature plays a crucial role in cooking. This foundational knowledge is essential for precise cooking.

2. **Practical Techniques**: Throughout the book, you'll find practical techniques and methods that you can apply in your kitchen immediately. From choosing the right cookware to preheating effectively, you'll learn how to create an environment that promotes even heat.

3. **Cooking Environments**: The book covers various cooking environments, from stovetop cooking to oven mastery and outdoor grilling. You'll discover how to achieve even heat on different platforms, allowing you to adapt your cooking methods to various recipes and ingredients.

4. **Troubleshooting**: Common cooking challenges can be frustrating, but this book equips you with troubleshooting tips. You'll learn how to identify and address issues such as hot spots and cold spots, overcooking, and undercooking. This knowledge will help you rescue dishes and ensure they turn out well.

5. **Timing and Temperature**: Achieving perfect timing is crucial in cooking, and it's closely tied to maintaining the right temperature. This book provides insights into timing and temperature control, including how to use thermometers and timers effectively.

6. **Recipes for Practice**: To put theory into practice, the book includes a collection of recipes. Each recipe is carefully crafted to highlight the importance of even heat. You'll have the opportunity to apply what you've learned and create delicious meals with step-by-step instructions and expert tips.

7. **Beyond the Kitchen**: Even heat extends beyond cooking.

The book explores applications of even heat in DIY projects, home brewing, and science experiments. You'll discover how the principles you've learned can be useful in various aspects of your life.

8. **Comprehensive Knowledge**: This book offers a comprehensive understanding of even heat, from its scientific foundations to practical applications. Whether you're a novice cook looking to improve your skills or an experienced chef seeking to refine your techniques, you'll find valuable insights within these pages.

9. **Consistency and Confidence**: By mastering even heat, you'll cook with greater consistency and confidence. Your dishes will turn out as expected, and you'll have the tools to adapt to new recipes and culinary challenges.

10. **Culinary Excellence**: Ultimately, this book aims to help you achieve culinary excellence. Whether you're cooking for yourself, your family, or guests, you'll be able to create dishes that are not only delicious but also beautifully cooked.

In summary, "Even Heat: The Key to Perfectly Cooked Dishes" is your trusted companion on a journey to culinary mastery. It empowers you with the knowledge, skills, and confidence needed to harness even heat in your cooking, ensuring that your dishes are consistently exceptional. Whether you're a passionate home cook or aspiring chef, this book is your key to unlocking the secrets of even heat and elevating your culinary skills.

Chapter Four

The Science of Heat

Understanding Heat Transfer

In the world of cooking, the mastery of heat is akin to wielding a painter's brush on a canvas. Just as an artist needs an intimate understanding of their tools and mediums to create a masterpiece, a skilled cook must comprehend the intricacies of heat to craft dishes that are nothing short of culinary art. This chapter, "The Science of Heat: Understanding Heat Transfer," serves as the foundation for your journey into the world of even heat, providing a comprehensive and exhaustive exploration of the principles and mechanisms governing the transfer of heat in cooking.

I. Introduction to the Science of Heat

Before delving into the specifics of heat transfer, it's essential to grasp the fundamental nature of heat itself. Heat, in its simplest definition, is a form of energy that flows from hotter objects to cooler ones. In the context of cooking, this energy is the driving force behind transformations in ingredients, leading to changes in flavor, texture, and appearance.

- **1.1 The Role of Heat in Cooking:** Heat is not just a cooking medium; it's the catalyst that triggers chemical reactions in food. These reactions are responsible for caramelization, browning, Maillard reactions, and other flavor-enhancing processes. Understanding the role of heat in cooking is the first step toward mastery.

II. Heat Transfer Mechanisms

Now, let's explore the mechanisms through which heat is transferred. Heat doesn't exist in isolation; it moves from one place to another by several methods, each with its unique characteristics and applications. In the culinary world, three primary mechanisms dominate:

1. Conduction

- **2.1 Definition:** Conduction is the transfer of heat through direct contact between two objects. In cooking, this typically involves the direct contact between a cooking vessel, such as a pan, and the food within it.

- **2.2 How Conduction Works:** When you place a pan on a burner, the heat from the burner is conducted through the pan and into the food. The heat flows from the hotter part (the burner) to the cooler part (the pan and food) until they reach equilibrium.

- **2.3 Practical Applications:** Conduction is the reason why you can sear a steak in a hot pan or simmer a soup in a pot. It's a fundamental heat transfer mechanism for stovetop cooking.

2. Convection

- **2.4 Definition:** Convection involves the transfer of heat through the movement of a fluid, such as air or liquid. In cooking, convection is often associated with ovens and water baths.

- **2.5 How Convection Works:** In an oven, for example, a fan circulates hot air, creating a convection current. This current carries heat to the food, ensuring even cooking. In sous vide cooking, water is heated and circulated to maintain a constant temperature.

- **2.6 Practical Applications:** Convection is responsible for even baking in ovens, roasting meats, and maintaining precise temperatures in sous vide cooking.

3. Radiation

- **2.7 Definition:** Radiation is the transfer of heat through electromagnetic waves, such as infrared radiation. It doesn't require a medium (unlike conduction and convection) and can travel through a vacuum.

- **2.8 How Radiation Works:** When you broil food in an oven or use a microwave, you're relying on radiation to heat your meal. In a broiler, infrared radiation from the heating element cooks the food's surface. In a microwave, microwaves (a type of radiation) excite water molecules, generating heat throughout the food.

- **2.9 Practical Applications:** Radiation is essential for browning, grilling, broiling, and microwaving food. It's particularly effective at creating crusts and surface browning.

III. Temperature: The Driving Force of Heat Transfer

Temperature is a fundamental concept in the science of heat. It's the measure of the average kinetic energy of particles in a substance. Understanding temperature and its role in cooking is paramount to achieving precise and consistent results.

- **3.1 Temperature Scales:** Temperature can be measured using various scales, with Celsius (°C) and Fahrenheit (°F) being the most common in cooking. In scientific contexts, the Kelvin (K) scale is often used.

- **3.2 Temperature Control:** The ability to control and adjust temperature is a cornerstone of successful cooking. Whether you're searing, simmering, or baking, knowing how to set and maintain the right temperature is essential.

- **3.3 Phase Transitions:** Temperature influences phase transitions, such as the transition from a solid to a liquid or from a liquid to a gas. These transitions play a crucial role in cooking, as they affect the texture and doneness of ingredients.

- **3.4 Thermal Equilibrium:** Achieving thermal equilibrium is the goal of most cooking processes. It occurs when all parts of a system (e.g., a piece of meat) reach the same temperature. This is when cooking is complete.

IV. Conductive Heat Transfer in Cooking

Now, let's dive deeper into conductive heat transfer, which is particularly relevant for stovetop cooking and various other culinary techniques.

- **4.1 Conductive Materials:** Not all materials conduct heat equally. Metals, such as copper and aluminum, are excellent conductors and are commonly used for cookware. Non-metal materials, like ceramics, can be poor conductors and may require special techniques.

- **4.2 The Cooking Vessel:** The choice of cooking vessel can significantly impact the rate of conductive heat transfer. Thin, lightweight pans heat up quickly but may result in uneven heating. Thick, heavy pans provide more even heat distribution but may take longer to heat.

- **4.3 Heat Capacity and Conductivity:** Heat capacity refers to the amount of heat a material can hold, while conductivity is its ability to transfer heat. Understanding these properties helps you select the right cookware for specific dishes and techniques.

- **4.4 Conductive Techniques:** Sautéing, frying, searing, and simmering are all examples of cooking techniques that rely on conductive heat transfer. Each technique requires a nuanced understanding of temperature and the conductive properties of the cooking vessel.

V. Convective Heat Transfer in Cooking

Convective heat transfer plays a pivotal role in techniques that involve ovens, water baths, and air circulation.

- **5.1 Forced Convection:** In cooking, forced convection involves the use of fans or pumps to circulate air or liquid. This method ensures that heat is distributed evenly, minimizing hot spots and cold spots.

- **5.2 Oven Cooking:** Convection ovens are designed to circulate hot air, creating a uniform temperature throughout the oven cavity. This even heat distribution is ideal for baking, roasting, and achieving consistent results.

- **5.3 Sous Vide Cooking:** Sous vide, a cooking method that involves immersing food in a precisely controlled water bath, relies on convection to maintain a constant and uniform temperature. This technique is renowned for its ability to achieve precise doneness.

VI. Radiative Heat Transfer in Cooking

Radiative heat transfer is responsible for browning, grilling, and some microwave cooking methods. Understanding how radiation works is essential for achieving specific culinary effects.

- **6.1 Browning Reactions:** Radiative heat transfer is often associated with browning reactions, such as caramelization and the Maillard reaction. These reactions require high temperatures and can impart complex flavors and appealing colors to food.

- **6.2 Broiling and Grilling:** Broilers and grills use radiant heat from heating elements or flames to cook food quickly at high temperatures. This method is particularly effective for creating crusts and searing.

- **6.3 Microwave Cooking:** Microwaves generate radiation, which excites water molecules in food, generating heat throughout the item. Understanding how microwaves work allows you to use this appliance effectively.

VII. Practical Considerations in Heat Transfer

In the real world of cooking, understanding heat transfer is not merely an academic exercise; it's a practical skill that leads to culinary success. This section explores the practical applications and considerations of heat transfer principles:

- **7.1 Heat Sources:** Different heat sources, such as gas burners, electric coils, open flames, and induction cooktops, have unique characteristics that influence how heat is transferred to your cookware and, subsequently, to your food.

- **7.2 Temperature Control:** Achieving precise temperature control is essential for various cooking techniques. You'll learn how to adjust your heat source to reach and maintain the desired temperature for your specific dish.

- **7.3 Heat Transfer Rates:** Various factors, including the type of cookware, its thickness, and the material's thermal conductivity, affect the rate of heat transfer. Understanding these factors helps you make informed decisions in the kitchen.

- **7.4 Food Properties:** Different ingredients and foods have varying thermal properties. Some foods conduct heat readily, while others insulate or resist heat. Recognizing these properties allows you to tailor your cooking methods accordingly.

- **7.5 Timing and Temperature Control:** Achieving perfect timing in cooking often relies on understanding temperature control. Knowing when to introduce heat, when to adjust it, and when to remove it is crucial for achieving consistent results.

- **7.6 Precision Cooking:** Techniques such as sous vide and precision baking demand precise temperature control. This section provides insights into how to maintain precise temperatures for extended periods.

VIII. Conclusion

As you journey through the intricacies of heat transfer in cooking, you'll gain a profound appreciation for the science that underpins every culinary creation. Understanding how heat moves, how temperature affects ingredients, and how to harness different heat transfer mechanisms will empower you to become a more versatile and confident cook.

Ultimately, this chapter serves as your gateway to mastering the art of even heat, which is at the heart of all great cooking. Armed with this knowledge, you'll approach your stovetop, oven, grill, and even your microwave with a deeper understanding of the transformative power of heat. You'll create dishes that are not only delicious but also beautifully and consistently cooked, elevating your culinary prowess to new heights.

In the chapters that follow, you'll build upon this foundation, delving into the practical applications of even heat in various cooking environments and techniques. With each page you turn, you'll take one step closer to becoming a true maestro in the culinary world, wielding the brush of heat with finesse to create culinary masterpieces in your own kitchen.

Chapter Five

The Role of Temperature in Cooking

Temperature is a fundamental factor in cooking, and understanding its role is essential for achieving precise and consistent results in the culinary arts. Whether you're searing a steak, baking a cake, or simmering a sauce, temperature plays a critical role in transforming raw ingredients into delicious dishes. In this exploration of the role of temperature in cooking, we will delve into its various facets, from the basic concepts to the nuanced applications that define culinary mastery.

I. Temperature: A Fundamental Measurement

Temperature is a measure of the average kinetic energy of particles in a substance. In simpler terms, it tells us how hot or cold something is. In cooking, we primarily use three temperature scales:

- **1.1 Celsius (°C):** The Celsius scale is based on the freezing point (0°C) and boiling point (100°C) of water at standard atmospheric pressure. It is widely used in most countries, except the United States.

- **1.2 Fahrenheit (°F):** The Fahrenheit scale, commonly used in the United States, is based on the freezing point (32°F) and boiling point (212°F) of water at standard atmospheric pressure.

- **1.3 Kelvin (K):** The Kelvin scale is an absolute temperature scale used in scientific contexts. It starts at absolute zero (0 K), the point at which all molecular motion ceases.

II. The Role of Temperature in Culinary Transformations

Temperature is the catalyst for various chemical and physical changes that occur during cooking. Here are some key ways temperature influences culinary transformations:

- **2.1 Melting:** Many ingredients, such as butter, chocolate, and sugar, undergo phase transitions when heated. Melting is the transformation from a solid to a liquid state. Precise control of melting temperatures is crucial in baking and confectionery.

- **2.2 Boiling and Evaporation:** Boiling occurs when a liquid reaches its boiling point, and vapor bubbles form throughout the liquid. Evaporation involves the conversion of a liquid to vapor at temperatures below its boiling point. Both processes are used in cooking to prepare various dishes, from pasta to soups.

- **2.3 Maillard Reaction:** The Maillard reaction is a complex chemical process that occurs between amino acids (found in proteins) and reducing sugars at elevated temperatures. It leads to the browning of foods and the development of rich, complex flavors. Precise temperature control is essential for achieving the desired Maillard reaction in dishes like seared steaks and roasted vegetables.

- **2.4 Caramelization:** Caramelization is the process of breaking down sugars at high temperatures to create a sweet, golden-brown syrup. This transformation is crucial in making caramel sauces, candies, and desserts.

- **2.5 Gelation:** Gelation occurs when proteins or starches in a liquid mixture form a gel-like structure as they heat and then cool. It is responsible for the texture of foods like custards, sauces, and gels.

- **2.6 Denaturation:** Proteins, such as those found in meat, eggs, and dairy products, undergo denaturation when exposed to heat. This process alters their structure, leading to changes in texture and doneness. Understanding the desired temperature for protein denaturation is key in techniques like sous vide cooking.

III. Precision Cooking and Temperature Control

The precise control of temperature is a hallmark of professional cooking and is increasingly accessible to home chefs. Understanding how to achieve and maintain the right temperature is critical for various culinary techniques:

- **3.1 Sous Vide Cooking:** Sous vide, a method of cooking food in vacuum-sealed bags at precise temperatures, relies on accurate temperature control to achieve specific levels of doneness. Whether you're aiming for a medium-rare steak or perfectly poached eggs, sous vide allows you to hit your target with precision.

- **3.2 Baking:** Baking involves cooking food in an enclosed space, such as an oven, at controlled temperatures. Precise temperature settings are vital for baking delicate pastries, bread, and cakes to perfection.

- **3.3 Searing:** Achieving the ideal sear on meat or fish requires precise temperature control. A searing hot pan ensures a flavorful crust without overcooking the interior.

- **3.4 Slow Cooking:** Slow-cooking methods, like braising and stewing, rely on low, steady temperatures over an extended period to tenderize tough cuts of meat and develop complex flavors.

- **3.5 Simmering:** Simmering is a gentle cooking technique that maintains a liquid at a temperature just below boiling. It's used for sauces, soups, and stews to meld flavors and ensure ingredients are thoroughly cooked.

IV. Temperature and Timing

Timing in cooking is closely linked to temperature. Knowing when to introduce heat, when to adjust it, and when to remove it is crucial for achieving consistent results. Timing considerations include:

- **4.1 Preheating:** Preheating ovens, pans, and grills to the desired cooking temperature ensures that food cooks evenly from the start. It's a foundational step for successful cooking.

- **4.2 Resting:** Allowing cooked food to rest after cooking is essential. Resting enables carryover cooking, where the

 M.A. GORRE

residual heat continues to cook the food even after it's re-
moved from the heat source. This ensures that the food is

Chapter Six

Conductive, Convective, and Radiant Heat

In the world of cooking, three primary mechanisms dominate the transfer of heat: conductive heat, convective heat, and radiant heat. Each of these mechanisms plays a distinct role in the culinary world, contributing to the art and science of preparing delicious dishes. Let's explore the characteristics, applications, and practical implications of these heat transfer methods:

I. Conductive Heat

1.1 Definition: Conductive heat transfer is the process by which heat moves through direct contact between two objects or substances. It occurs when one object, typically a solid, transfers its thermal energy to another object in contact with it.

1.2 How Conductive Heat Works:

When you place a pan on a stovetop burner, for example, the burner heats the bottom of the pan. The heat is conducted through the metal of the pan and into the food. The heat flows from the hotter part (the burner) to the cooler part (the pan and food) until they reach equilibrium.

1.3 Practical Applications:

Conductive heat transfer is fundamental in cooking. It's responsible for:

- Searing steaks in a hot pan

- Frying foods in oil

- Simmering sauces in a pot

- Baking cookies on a baking sheet

II. Convective Heat

2.1 Definition: Convective heat transfer occurs when heat is transferred through the movement of a fluid, such as air or liquid. Convection involves the bulk movement of the fluid itself, which carries heat from one location to another.

2.2 How Convective Heat Works:

In an oven, for example, a fan circulates hot air throughout the oven cavity. This circulating air carries heat to the food, ensuring even cooking. In sous vide cooking, water is heated and circulated to maintain a constant temperature around the food.

2.3 Practical Applications:

Convective heat transfer is essential in cooking techniques such as:

- Baking bread and pastries in an oven

- Roasting meats to perfection

- Achieving consistent temperatures in sous vide cooking

- Maintaining uniform heat in convection ovens

III. Radiant Heat

3.1 Definition: Radiant heat transfer is the process of heat being transferred through electromagnetic waves, such as infrared radiation. Unlike conductive and convective heat, radiant heat doesn't require a medium (like air or water) to transfer heat; it can travel through a vacuum.

3.2 How Radiant Heat Works:

Radiant heat is often associated with high-temperature sources, such as broilers, grills, and microwave ovens. In a broiler, for instance, infrared radiation emitted by the heating element cooks the food's surface. In a microwave oven, microwaves (a type of radiation) excite water molecules, generating heat throughout the food.

3.3 Practical Applications:

Radiant heat transfer is integral in cooking for:

- Browning and searing meats on grills

- Broiling dishes in the oven for surface browning

- Microwaving food to heat and cook it quickly

- Achieving crusts and surface browning in baking and roasting

IV. Combining Heat Transfer Methods

In many cooking scenarios, these three heat transfer mechanisms work together to create the desired culinary outcomes. For example:

- When roasting a chicken in the oven, convective heat from the circulating hot air cooks the meat evenly, while radiant heat from the oven's heating element provides surface browning.

- In sous vide cooking, precise control of temperature (conductive) is combined with convection (circulating water) to maintain uniform cooking throughout.

- When stir-frying in a hot wok, conductive heat from the wok's surface sears the ingredients, while convective heat from the moving air ensures even cooking.

V. Temperature and Control

Understanding and controlling the temperature of these heat transfer mechanisms is a fundamental skill in cooking:

- For conductive heat, precise temperature control of stovetop burners or ovens is crucial for achieving desired results.

- In convective cooking, understanding the temperature settings of ovens and the circulation of hot air helps ensure even cooking.

- Radiant heat sources, like grills and broilers, often involve controlling the distance between the heat source and the food to achieve the desired level of browning and cooking.

VI. Practical Considerations

- **Cookware Selection:** The choice of cookware can significantly impact the rate of conductive heat transfer. Thick, heavy pans distribute heat more evenly, while thin pans may lead to hot spots.

- **Flavor Development:** Each heat transfer method can influence the flavor of dishes. For instance, the Maillard reaction, responsible for browning and flavor development, occurs primarily through radiant and conductive heat.

- **Timing:** Understanding when to introduce and adjust heat during the cooking process is crucial for achieving the desired doneness and texture in dishes.

- **Combining Techniques:** Many recipes involve a combination of heat transfer methods. Knowing how to leverage these methods effectively can lead to culinary success.

In summary, conductive, convective, and radiant heat transfer are the fundamental mechanisms that bring ingredients to life in the culinary world. Mastering these methods and understanding how they interact is essential for achieving precise and consistent cooking results, whether you're searing a steak, baking bread, or grilling vegetables. It's through the skillful use of these heat transfer mechanisms that chefs and home cooks alike create delicious and beautifully cooked dishes that delight the palate.

Chapter Seven

The Cooking Basics

Choosing the Right Cookware

Cookware is the foundation of every kitchen, and selecting the right pots, pans, and utensils is essential for successful cooking. The choice of cookware can significantly impact your ability to achieve even heat distribution, control, and the desired results in your dishes. In this guide, we will explore the basics of choosing the right cookware to set you up for culinary success.

I. Understanding Cookware Materials

Cookware comes in a wide variety of materials, each with its unique properties. Understanding these materials is crucial when making your selection:

1. Stainless Steel:

- **Advantages:** Stainless steel is durable, non-reactive with food, and resistant to staining and rust. It's an excellent choice for searing, browning, and deglazing.

- **Considerations:** Stainless steel does not conduct heat as evenly as some other materials, so it often has an aluminum or copper core to improve heat distribution.

2. Nonstick:

- **Advantages:** Nonstick coatings, like Teflon, make cooking and cleaning a breeze. They're ideal for low-fat cooking and delicate items like eggs and pancakes.

- **Considerations:** Nonstick pans should be used with care to avoid scratching the coating. High heat can damage nonstick surfaces, so they are not suitable for searing or broiling.

3. Cast Iron:

- **Advantages:** Cast iron retains and distributes heat exceptionally well. It's ideal for frying, baking, and slow-cooking, and it can develop a natural nonstick surface (seasoning) over time.

- **Considerations:** Cast iron requires proper seasoning and maintenance to prevent rust. It's heavy and may take longer to heat up.

4. Copper:

- **Advantages:** Copper is an excellent conductor of heat, providing precise temperature control. It's favored by professional chefs for tasks that require quick and precise adjustments.

- **Considerations:** Copper cookware often has a stainless steel or tin lining, as pure copper can react with acidic foods. It can also be expensive.

5. Aluminum:

- **Advantages:** Aluminum is an excellent heat conductor and is often used in clad cookware with other materials like stainless steel. It heats up quickly and distributes heat evenly.

- **Considerations:** Uncoated aluminum can react with acidic foods, so it's usually anodized or coated.

II. Considerations for Cookware Selection

When choosing cookware for your kitchen, several factors should be considered:

1. Cooking Method:

- Different cooking methods require specific types of cookware. For instance, a heavy-bottomed stainless steel pan is excellent for searing, while a nonstick skillet is ideal for omelets.

2. Heat Conductivity:

- Consider how evenly and efficiently the material conducts heat. Even heat distribution helps prevent hot spots and ensures consistent cooking.

3. Durability:

- The durability of your cookware is essential. High-quality materials and construction can ensure that your pots and pans last for years.

4. Maintenance:

- Some cookware, like cast iron, requires regular seasoning and maintenance. Others, like stainless steel, are relatively low-maintenance.

5. Compatibility:

- Ensure that your cookware is compatible with your cooking

appliances, such as induction stovetops or ovens.

6. Price Range:

- Cookware comes in a wide range of price points. Consider your budget and invest in quality pieces that will serve you well.

III. Essential Cookware Pieces

Every kitchen should have a few essential cookware pieces to cover a variety of cooking tasks:

1. Skillet/Frying Pan:

- An all-purpose skillet is versatile and suitable for frying, sautéing, searing, and even baking.

2. Saucepan:

- A saucepan is great for making sauces, heating liquids, and cooking grains.

3. Stockpot:

- A stockpot is ideal for making soups, stews, and large batches of pasta.

4. Dutch Oven:

- A Dutch oven is a versatile, heavy-duty pot that can be used for braising, roasting, frying, and baking.

5. Baking Sheet:

- A baking sheet is essential for roasting vegetables, baking cookies, and many other oven-related tasks.

6. Nonstick Pan:

- A nonstick pan is convenient for low-fat cooking and delicate foods.

7. Cast Iron Skillet:

- A cast iron skillet is excellent for searing, frying, baking, and more.

IV. Care and Maintenance

Proper care and maintenance of your cookware can extend its lifespan and performance:

- Follow the manufacturer's instructions for cleaning and seasoning cast iron cookware.

- Avoid using metal utensils in nonstick pans to prevent scratching.

- Hand wash your cookware when possible to preserve its finish and nonstick properties.

- Regularly check for signs of wear and tear, such as peeling nonstick coating or loose handles, and replace damaged cookware.

In conclusion, choosing the right cookware is essential for achieving success in the kitchen. By considering your cooking style, heat conductivity preferences, and maintenance requirements, you can build a collection of cookware that serves you well and enhances your culinary adventures. With the right tools at your disposal, you'll be well-equipped to explore a world of delicious recipes and culinary creativity.

Chapter Eight

Properly Preheating Your Cookware

Properly preheating your cookware is a fundamental step in achieving consistent and delicious cooking results. Whether you're searing a steak, sautéing vegetables, or baking a cake, preheating ensures even heat distribution, prevents sticking, and contributes to the development of desirable flavors and textures. In this guide, we'll explore the importance of preheating and how to do it effectively for various types of cookware.

I. Why Preheat Your Cookware

Preheating your cookware is crucial for several reasons:

1. Even Heat Distribution:

- Preheating allows the entire surface of the cookware to reach the desired temperature. This helps prevent hot spots and ensures that food cooks evenly.

2. Prevents Sticking:

- When you preheat a pan or skillet, it creates a nonstick surface through the Maillard reaction, which forms a layer that helps food release more easily.

3. Flavor Development:

- Preheating is essential for achieving caramelization and the Maillard reaction, which contribute to the development of complex flavors and appealing colors in food.

II. How to Properly Preheat Cookware

The preheating process varies depending on the type of cookware you're using. Here are some guidelines for preheating different types of cookware:

1. Preheating Stainless Steel and Cast Iron Cookware:

- Place the empty pan on the burner over medium to medium-high heat.

- Allow the pan to heat for several minutes until it's uniformly hot. You can test the readiness by sprinkling a few drops of water into the pan. If the water droplets sizzle and evaporate almost instantly, the pan is likely hot enough.

- Once the pan is adequately preheated, add your cooking oil or fat and swirl it around to coat the bottom evenly.

- Allow the oil or fat to heat for a brief additional period (around 30 seconds) before adding your ingredients.

2. Preheating Nonstick Cookware:

- Preheating nonstick pans requires extra care to avoid overheating, which can damage the nonstick coating.

- Place the empty nonstick pan on the burner over low to medium heat.

- Allow the pan to heat for a short time, usually 1 to 2 minutes.

- Once the pan feels warm to the touch, add your cooking oil or fat and proceed with your recipe.

3. Preheating Oven for Baking:
- Preheating the oven is essential for baking and roasting.

- Set your oven to the desired temperature and allow it to preheat for at least 10-15 minutes. Some ovens may require longer preheating times.

- Baking and roasting temperatures vary depending on the recipe, so always follow the specific instructions provided.

4. Preheating Grills and Outdoor Cookware:
- Preheating grills and outdoor cookware, such as barbecue grills or cast iron griddles, is essential for achieving the right cooking temperature and preventing sticking.

- Follow the manufacturer's instructions for preheating your specific grill or cookware.

- Allow sufficient time for the grill or cookware to reach the desired temperature before cooking your food.

III. Tips for Effective Preheating

To ensure effective preheating, consider these additional tips:

1. Use the Right Temperature:
- Choose the appropriate heat setting for your cookware and

recipe. For example, searing typically requires high heat, while delicate sautéing may be done over medium heat.

2. Be Patient:

- Proper preheating takes time. Rushing this step can result in uneven cooking and less desirable outcomes.

3. Test with Water:

- If you're uncertain whether your pan is hot enough, you can use the water droplet test. Simply sprinkle a few drops of water into the pan. If the water sizzles and evaporates rapidly, the pan is ready.

4. Don't Overheat Nonstick Pans:

- Overheating nonstick pans can damage the nonstick coating. Always use low to medium heat when preheating nonstick cookware.

5. Monitor the Temperature:

- If you're using a thermometer, such as an infrared thermometer or an oven thermometer, you can verify the temperature of your cookware or oven to ensure accuracy.

In conclusion, properly preheating your cookware is a fundamental step in achieving culinary success. It promotes even heat distribution, prevents sticking, and enhances the flavor and texture of your dishes. By following the guidelines and tips provided for different types of cookware, you'll be well-equipped to preheat effectively and embark on a journey to create delicious and beautifully cooked meals.

Chapter Nine

Essential Cooking Techniques

Mastering essential cooking techniques is the foundation of becoming a skilled and confident cook. These techniques provide you with the knowledge and skills needed to prepare a wide range of dishes with precision and creativity. Here are some essential cooking techniques that every home cook should learn:

1. **Searing:**

   - Searing involves cooking food quickly over high heat to create a flavorful, caramelized crust. It's commonly used for steaks, chops, and seafood.

   - Tips: Pat food dry before searing, use a hot pan with oil, and avoid overcrowding the pan.

2. **Sautéing:**

   - Sautéing is a method of cooking food quickly in a small amount of oil or butter over high heat. It's perfect for vegetables, mushrooms, and thinly sliced meats.

- Tips: Keep the pan and food in motion to prevent sticking and achieve even cooking.

3. Roasting:

- Roasting involves cooking food in the oven, typically at high temperatures. It's great for meats, poultry, and vegetables.

- Tips: Use a roasting rack to allow air circulation, and season the food with herbs and spices for flavor.

4. Grilling:

- Grilling is the process of cooking food over an open flame or on a grill. It's excellent for steaks, burgers, chicken, and vegetables.

- Tips: Preheat the grill, oil the grates to prevent sticking, and practice proper timing for doneness.

5. Braising:

- Braising is a slow-cooking method that involves searing food, then simmering it in a flavorful liquid. It's ideal for tough cuts of meat.

- Tips: Choose a heavy pot with a tight-fitting lid, and use a flavorful liquid like broth or wine.

6. Boiling and Blanching:

- Boiling involves cooking food in rapidly boiling water, while blanching briefly boils food before quickly cooling it. Both techniques are used for pasta, vegetables, and seafood.

- Tips: Use plenty of salt in boiling water, and have an ice bath ready for blanching to stop cooking and retain color.

7. Simmering:

- Simmering is gentle boiling where food cooks slowly in a liquid at a lower temperature. It's perfect for soups, stews, and sauces.

- Tips: Maintain a consistent low heat to prevent boiling, and periodically skim off impurities from the surface.

8. Baking:

- Baking involves cooking food in an oven using dry heat. It's used for bread, pastries, cakes, and casseroles.

- Tips: Preheat the oven for even cooking, and use the correct temperature and baking time from recipes.

9. Frying:

- Frying is cooking food by submerging it in hot oil. There are two primary methods: deep frying (fully submerging) and shallow frying (partially submerging).

- Tips: Use a thermometer to monitor oil temperature, and drain fried foods on paper towels to remove excess oil.

10. Poaching:

- Poaching involves gently simmering food in liquid, typically water or broth. It's often used for delicate items like eggs and fish.
- Tips: Keep the poaching liquid at a low simmer, and use a flavorful liquid or aromatics for added taste.

11. Stir-Frying:

- Stir-frying is a quick-cooking method that involves cooking small pieces of food in a hot pan or wok with constant stirring. It's common in Asian cuisine.

- Tips: Prep ingredients ahead of time, and cook over high heat while continuously tossing or stirring.

12. Deglazing:

- Deglazing is the process of adding liquid (e.g., wine or broth) to a hot pan to loosen and incorporate flavorful browned bits (fond) from seared or sautéed food.

- Tips: Use a flavorful liquid, scrape the pan with a wooden spoon, and reduce the liquid to make a sauce.

13. Mincing and Chopping:

- Mincing involves cutting food into very small, uniform pieces, while chopping produces larger, irregular pieces. Both are essential for preparing ingredients like garlic, onions, and herbs.

- Tips: Use a sharp knife and practice proper cutting techniques to achieve desired results.

14. Whisking and Emulsifying:

- Whisking combines ingredients by vigorously stirring with a whisk. Emulsifying is a specific type of whisking used to combine two immiscible liquids, like oil and vinegar in salad dressings.

- Tips: Whisk in a consistent pattern to incorporate air, and add oil slowly when emulsifying to prevent separation.

15. Seasoning:

- Properly seasoning food with salt, pepper, herbs, and spices is a fundamental technique that enhances flavor in every dish.

- Tips: Taste as you season and adjust gradually to avoid over-seasoning.

16. Measuring:

- Precise measuring of ingredients is essential for baking and cooking. It ensures consistency and accurate results.

- Tips: Use proper measuring tools, level dry ingredients, and measure liquids at eye level.

17. Tasting and Adjusting:

- Regularly tasting your dishes as you cook allows you to adjust seasoning, acidity, and other flavors to achieve the desired taste.
- Tips: Keep clean spoons or tasting utensils on hand, and make gradual adjustments to avoid overcorrection.

Mastering these essential cooking techniques will empower you to explore a wide range of recipes and cuisines, and it's the first step toward becoming a confident and skilled home cook. With practice and experimentation, you'll develop the ability to create delicious meals that delight your taste buds and those of your loved ones.

Chapter Ten

Stovetop Cooking Mastering the Gas Stove

A gas stove is a versatile and popular choice for cooking in many kitchens. Mastering the use of a gas stove allows you to have precise control over heat levels and perform a wide range of cooking techniques. In this guide, we'll explore the key components of a gas stove and provide tips and techniques for cooking effectively.

I. Understanding the Gas Stove Components

Before you start cooking, it's essential to understand the components of a gas stove:

1. Burners:

- Gas stoves typically have multiple burners, each with its control knob. The burners provide the heat source for cooking.

2. Control Knobs:

- Control knobs are used to adjust the flame intensity on each burner. They allow you to increase or decrease the heat as needed.

3. Burner Grates:

- Burner grates provide a stable surface for your pots and pans. They also help distribute heat evenly.

4. Ignition System:

- Many gas stoves have an ignition system that uses an electric spark to light the gas when you turn the control knob.

II. Tips for Using a Gas Stove

Here are some essential tips for effectively using a gas stove:

1. Lighting the Burners:

- To light a gas burner, turn the corresponding control knob counterclockwise to the "light" or "ignite" position. If your stove has an electric ignition, you'll hear a clicking sound as it sparks to ignite the gas.

- Hold the knob down for a few seconds after the flame ignites to ensure it stays lit.

2. Adjusting Flame Intensity:

- Use the control knobs to adjust the flame intensity. Turn the knob counterclockwise to increase the flame and clockwise to decrease it.

- Start with a high flame for boiling or searing and lower it for simmering or gentle cooking.

3. Using Different Burners:

- Depending on your stove, different burners may have varying heat outputs. Use the appropriate burner for the cooking task. For example, use the back burners for simmering and the front burners for high-heat cooking.

4. Cookware Selection:

- Choose cookware that matches the size of the burner. Using pots and pans that are too small or too large for the burner can result in uneven cooking.

5. Flame Control:

- Be cautious when adjusting the flame intensity, especially when using high heat. Rapidly changing the flame level can lead to uneven cooking or boil-overs.

III. Common Cooking Techniques on a Gas Stove

A gas stove is suitable for various cooking techniques. Here are some common ones:

1. Searing:

- For a perfect sear on steaks or other meats, preheat a heavy skillet over high heat until it's very hot, then add the meat.

2. Sauteing:

- Sauteing involves cooking food quickly in a small amount of oil or butter in a wide, shallow pan over medium-high heat.

3. Simmering:

- To simmer, use a low flame to maintain a gentle, steady boil for soups, stews, and sauces. Use the back burners for simmering to prevent scorching.

4. Boiling:

- Bring a large pot of water to a rolling boil on high heat for pasta, vegetables, or potatoes.

5. Stir-Frying:

- Stir-frying is a high-heat cooking method that involves quickly cooking small pieces of food in a wok or skillet. Use the highest flame setting.

6. Grilling:

- If your gas stove has a grill attachment or you have a stovetop grill pan, you can mimic grilling by using a high flame.

IV. Safety Considerations

Safety is paramount when using a gas stove:

1. Ventilation:

- Ensure that your kitchen is well-ventilated to prevent the buildup of gas fumes. Use a range hood or open a window if necessary.

2. Gas Odor:

- If you detect a strong gas odor when using your stove, turn off the burners, open windows, and do not use the stove until the issue is resolved.

3. Flame Safety:

- Be attentive when cooking, and never leave a gas stove unattended while it's in use.

4. Carbon Monoxide Detector:

- Consider installing a carbon monoxide detector in your kitchen to alert you to any gas leaks.

5. Regular Maintenance:

- Periodically inspect your gas stove for any signs of wear or damage, and have it serviced as needed to ensure safe operation.

Mastering the use of a gas stove can significantly enhance your cooking skills. With proper control of flame intensity and a good understanding of cooking techniques, you'll be able to prepare a wide range of dishes with precision and confidence. Always prioritize safety and maintain your gas stove to ensure its reliable performance in your kitchen.

Chapter Eleven

Electric Stovetops: Tips and Tricks

Electric stovetops are a common choice in many kitchens, offering consistent and even heat for cooking. To make the most of your electric stovetop, it's essential to understand how it works and implement some helpful tips and tricks. In this guide, we'll explore the key features of electric stovetops and provide you with practical advice to improve your cooking experience.

I. Understanding Electric Stovetop Components

Before diving into tips and tricks, let's familiarize ourselves with the components of an electric stovetop:

1. Heating Elements:

- Electric stovetops have one or more heating elements, usually made of coiled metal or a smooth ceramic glass surface.

2. Control Knobs or Touch Controls:

- Control knobs or touch controls are used to adjust the heat level of each heating element. They allow you to increase or decrease the temperature as needed.

3. Indicator Lights:

- Indicator lights may be present to show when a heating element is active or hot. Some models have residual heat indicators to warn when a surface is still hot even after it's turned off.

II. Tips and Tricks for Cooking on Electric Stovetops

Here are some tips and tricks to help you make the most of your electric stovetop:

1. Preheat Pans:

- Preheat your cookware before adding ingredients. This helps ensure even cooking and prevents sticking.

- For best results, use pans with a flat, heavy-bottomed base to distribute heat evenly.

2. Match Pot and Burner Sizes:

- Match the size of your pots and pans to the heating element. Using a pot that's too small or too large can result in inefficient cooking and longer cooking times.

3. Use Flat-Bottomed Cookware:

- Flat-bottomed pots and pans make direct contact with the heating element, maximizing heat transfer and efficiency.

4. Adjust Heat Gradually:

- Electric stovetops can take a little time to change temperature. Adjust the heat gradually to avoid overshooting your desired cooking temperature.

5. Simmering and Low Heat:

- For simmering or cooking at low heat, consider using a heat diffuser or simmer ring to spread the heat evenly and prevent scorching.

6. Cookware Material:

- Choose cookware that is compatible with electric stovetops. Stainless steel, cast iron, and flat-bottomed aluminum pans work well.

7. Avoid Excessive Movement:

- Minimize moving pots and pans around while cooking. Frequent stirring or repositioning can cause uneven heating.

8. Optimize Pan Size:

- Use pans that match the size of the heating element. This ensures that the entire bottom surface receives even heat.

9. Keep Cookware Clean:

- Clean your cookware regularly to prevent the buildup of residue, which can affect heat transfer and cooking performance.

10. Use Cookware Lids:

- When appropriate, cover your cookware with a lid to trap heat and speed up cooking, especially when boiling water or simmering.

11. Boiling Water:

- When boiling water, use a kettle to bring it to a boil faster. Then, transfer it to a pot on the stovetop for further cooking.

12. Maintain a Steady Heat:

- For foods that require a steady, consistent heat, such as custards or sauces, use a double boiler or a heat diffuser to prevent scorching.

13. Cast Iron Griddle:

- If you have a smooth electric stovetop, consider using a cast iron griddle for pancakes, grilled sandwiches, and more. It provides even heating.

III. Safety Considerations

Safety is essential when using electric stovetops:

1. Turn Off After Use:

- Always turn off the heating elements when you're finished cooking.

2. Use Caution with Glass Cooktops:

- Glass cooktops can retain heat even after being turned off. Be cautious and avoid placing items on the surface immediately after cooking.

3. Keep Cooktop Clean:

- Regularly clean your electric stovetop to prevent the buildup of food debris, which can affect heating efficiency.

4. Childproof Controls:

- If you have young children, consider childproofing the control knobs or using stove knob covers to prevent accidental activation.

Mastering the use of your electric stovetop takes practice, but with these tips and tricks, you'll be able to cook with precision and efficiency. Remember to match your cookware to the heating elements, adjust heat gradually, and maintain a clean and well-maintained stovetop for optimal cooking results.

Chapter Twelve

Induction Cooking: Precision and Control

Induction cooking is known for its precision, speed, and energy efficiency. It utilizes electromagnetic technology to heat cookware directly, offering precise temperature control and fast heating. In this guide, we'll explore the benefits of induction cooking and provide tips to maximize its precision and control.

I. How Induction Cooking Works

Induction cooking relies on electromagnetic induction to generate heat. Here's how it works:

1. **Magnetic Fields:** Induction cooktops contain copper coils that produce alternating magnetic fields when electricity flows through them.

2. **Cookware Compatibility:** To work with induction, your cookware must have a magnetic bottom. Induction-compatible cookware typically includes stainless steel, cast iron, and some types of enameled cookware.

3. **Magnetic Interaction:** When you place induction-compatible cookware on the cooktop, the magnetic field induces an electric current within the cookware itself.

4. **Heat Generation:** The induced electric current generates heat directly within the cookware, heating it and the food or liquid inside.

II. Benefits of Induction Cooking

Induction cooking offers several advantages, including:

1. **Precise Temperature Control:** Induction cooktops allow you to adjust heat levels with great precision, ensuring accurate cooking and preventing overcooking or burning.

2. **Speed:** Induction heats cookware and food rapidly, reducing cooking times and saving energy.

3. **Energy Efficiency:** Since heat is generated directly in the cookware, there's minimal heat loss to the surrounding environment, making induction cooking highly efficient.

4. **Safety:** Induction cooktops remain cool to the touch, reducing the risk of burns. They also feature automatic shutoff mechanisms for added safety.

5. **Easy Cleanup:** Induction cooktops have a smooth surface that is easy to clean, as spills are less likely to burn onto the cooktop.

III. Tips for Maximizing Precision and Control

To get the most out of induction cooking, follow these tips:

1. Use Proper Cookware:

- Ensure your cookware is compatible with induction cooking by checking if it has a magnetic bottom. Stainless steel and cast iron are excellent choices.

2. Match Cookware Size to Burner:

- Use cookware that matches the size of the induction burner. This ensures efficient and even heating.

3. Precise Temperature Settings:

- Take advantage of the precise temperature control by adjusting settings to the specific cooking needs of your recipe.

4. Experiment and Learn:

- Spend time experimenting with different heat levels and settings to understand how your induction cooktop responds to various cooking techniques.

5. Avoid Excessive Movement:

- Minimize moving cookware around once it's placed on the cooktop. Induction responds quickly to adjustments, so there's no need for excessive stirring or repositioning.

6. Use Cookware Lids:

- When appropriate, use lids on pots and pans to trap heat, reduce cooking times, and prevent moisture loss.

7. Keep Cooktop Clean:

- Regularly clean your induction cooktop to ensure efficient heat transfer. Clean up spills promptly to prevent them from becoming stubborn stains.

8. Be Mindful of Potentially Damaging Items:

- Avoid placing items like aluminum foil or empty cookware on the cooktop, as they can disrupt the magnetic field and potentially damage the cooktop.

9. Practice Safety:

- Familiarize yourself with the safety features of your induction cooktop, such as automatic shutoff, and use them as needed.

10. Get Familiar with Cookware Sensitivity:

- Induction cooktops can be sensitive to changes in cookware placement. Learn how quickly your cookware responds to adjustments in temperature settings.

IV. Safety Considerations

While induction cooking is generally safe, it's important to be aware of potential safety considerations:

1. **Burn Risk:** While the cooktop itself remains cool, the cookware and its contents can become very hot. Exercise caution when handling hot pots and pans.

2. **Electromagnetic Sensitivity:** Some electronic devices and pacemakers may be sensitive to the electromagnetic fields generated by induction cooktops. Consult with a medical professional if you have concerns.

3. **Cookware Placement:** Be mindful of where you place cookware on the cooktop to avoid disrupting the magnetic field.

Induction cooking offers unparalleled precision and control in the kitchen. With the right cookware and a good understanding of its features, you can take full advantage of this efficient and convenient cooking method to prepare delicious meals with ease.

Chapter Thirteen

Oven Mastery

Conventional vs. Convection Ovens, Positioning and Rack Placement, Baking, Roasting, and Broiling Techniques

Mastering your oven is a fundamental skill for any home cook. Ovens are versatile appliances that allow you to bake, roast, broil, and more. In this comprehensive guide, we'll explore the differences between conventional and convection ovens, discuss the importance of positioning and rack placement, and delve into essential techniques for baking, roasting, and broiling. By the end of this guide, you'll have the knowledge and confidence to harness the full potential of your oven.

I. Conventional vs. Convection Ovens

Before we dive into techniques, it's essential to understand the key differences between conventional and convection ovens:

1. Conventional Ovens:

- In a conventional oven, heat is generated by one or more heating elements, typically located at the bottom and top of the oven.

- Hot air rises naturally, creating a temperature difference between the top and bottom. This can result in uneven cooking.

2. Convection Ovens:

- Convection ovens have an additional feature—a fan. This fan circulates hot air throughout the oven, ensuring even and consistent heat distribution.

- As a result, convection ovens cook food faster and more evenly than conventional ovens.

II. Positioning and Rack Placement

The way you position your oven racks can significantly impact your cooking results. Here are some essential tips:

1. Center Rack Position:

- For most baking and roasting tasks, place the rack in the center position. This ensures even heat distribution around your food.

2. Upper Rack Position:

- Use the upper rack position for broiling or when you want to brown the top of a dish quickly. Keep a close eye on food when broiling to prevent burning.

3. Lower Rack Position:

- The lower rack position is suitable for baking items like bread or pizza directly on the oven's bottom to achieve a crisp crust.

4. Multiple Racks:

- When using multiple racks, stagger them to allow heat to circulate freely. Leave enough space between pans for good air circulation.

5. Baking Stones and Baking Sheets:

- For items like pizza or artisan bread, consider using baking stones or baking sheets on the oven's bottom rack to mimic the intense heat of a pizza oven.

III. Baking Techniques

Baking is a fundamental cooking technique used for a wide range of dishes, from cakes and cookies to casseroles and bread. Here are some key baking tips:

1. Preheating:

- Always preheat your oven to the desired temperature before placing your food inside. This ensures consistent cooking from the start.

2. Baking Pans:

- Choose the right baking pan for your recipe. Different recipes may call for metal, glass, or ceramic pans. Adjust baking times and temperatures accordingly.

3. Oven Thermometer:

- Use an oven thermometer to verify the accuracy of your oven's temperature settings. Oven thermostats can sometimes be slightly off.

4. Rotating Pans:

- For even baking, consider rotating your pans halfway through the baking time. This helps prevent uneven browning.

5. Oven Light:

- Use the oven light to check on your food's progress without opening the oven door. Frequent opening and closing can affect temperature consistency.

IV. Roasting Techniques

Roasting is a cooking method that involves cooking food uncovered in the oven, usually at higher temperatures. It's commonly used for meats and vegetables. Here's how to master roasting:

1. Seasoning:

- Season your meat or vegetables generously with salt, pepper, and any desired herbs and spices. Let them sit at room temperature for about 30 minutes before roasting for better flavor absorption.

2. Roasting Pan:

- Use a roasting pan with a rack to elevate the food above any drippings. This allows heat to circulate evenly and promotes even browning.

3. Temperature Control:

- For meats, use a meat thermometer to monitor the internal temperature. Roast to your desired level of doneness. A probe thermometer is handy for this purpose.

4. Resting:

- After roasting, let meat rest for a few minutes before carving. This allows the juices to redistribute, resulting in a juicier, more tender dish.

V. Broiling Techniques

Broiling is a cooking method that exposes food to high, direct heat from the oven's broiler element. It's great for quickly browning the tops of dishes. Here's how to use your broiler effectively:

1. Broiler Pan:

- Use a broiler pan or a similar oven-safe dish to hold your food. The slotted pan allows excess fat and juices to drip away.

2. Preheating:

- Preheat the broiler for a few minutes before placing your food inside. This ensures that the broiler element is at its maximum heat.

3. Adjust Rack Position:

- When broiling, use the upper rack position. Keep the food relatively close to the broiler element, but not too close to prevent burning.

4. Watching Closely:

- Broiling is a quick process, so keep a close eye on your food. It can go from perfectly browned to burned in a matter of seconds.

5. Flipping:

- If necessary, flip or turn your food to ensure even browning on both sides.

VI. Oven Maintenance

Proper oven maintenance is crucial for consistent cooking results and safety. Here are some maintenance tips:

1. Regular Cleaning:

- Clean your oven regularly, especially after spills or drips. Built-up food residue can affect cooking performance and even cause smoke or odors.

2. Self-Cleaning Function:

- Many ovens have a self-cleaning function. Use it periodically to burn off any stubborn residues. Follow the manufacturer's instructions.

3. Door Seal:

- Check the oven door seal for signs of wear or damage. A damaged seal can result in heat loss and uneven cooking.

4. Replace Oven Light Bulb:

- If the oven light bulb burns out, replace it promptly so you can monitor your food's progress.

5. Professional Maintenance:

- If you encounter issues with temperature consistency or other problems, consider having your oven professionally serviced.

By mastering these techniques and understanding the nuances of conventional and convection ovens, you'll have the knowledge and skills to confidently create a wide range of dishes. Whether you're baking delicate pastries, roasting succulent meats, or broiling perfectly golden cheese, your oven will become a trusted ally in your culinary adventur

Chapter Fourteen

Grilling and Outdoor Cooking

Achieving Even Heat on the Grill, Smoking and Slow Cooking, Maintaining Heat in Outdoor Ovens

Grilling and outdoor cooking are timeless culinary traditions that bring people together over delicious meals and the wonderful aroma of food sizzling over an open flame. Whether you're a seasoned grill master or just getting started with outdoor cooking, this comprehensive guide will equip you with the knowledge and techniques needed to achieve even heat on the grill, explore the art of smoking and slow cooking, and maintain heat in outdoor ovens. Let's dive into the world of outdoor culinary adventures.

I. Achieving Even Heat on the Grill

Grilling is all about getting that perfect sear and smoky flavor on your food. Achieving even heat on the grill is key to ensuring that every bite is cooked to perfection. Here's how to do it:

1. Preheating:

- Preheat your grill with all burners on high for at least 15-20 minutes before cooking. This allows the grates to get hot and helps eliminate any food residues.

2. Two-Zone Grilling:

- Create two zones on your grill—direct and indirect heat. On a gas grill, this involves turning off one set of burners after preheating. On a charcoal grill, arrange the coals to create a hot zone and a cooler zone.

3. Use a Grill Thermometer:

- Invest in a good-quality grill thermometer to monitor the temperature accurately. Grill temperatures can vary from spot to spot.

4. Adjust the Grill Grates:

- Adjust the height of your grill grates. For high-heat searing, position them close to the flames. For slower cooking or indirect grilling, raise the grates.

5. Lid On vs. Lid Off:

- Keep the grill lid on for foods that require indirect heat or slow cooking, like roasts or whole chickens. Leave it off for direct grilling, such as burgers and steaks.

6. Flip and Rotate:

- Flip and rotate your food as needed to ensure even cooking. Use long-handled tongs or a spatula to avoid losing precious grill marks.

II. Smoking and Slow Cooking

Smoking and slow cooking take outdoor cooking to the next level, infusing your food with delicious smoky flavors and tenderness. Here's how to get started:

1. Smoking Basics:

- Smoking involves cooking food at low temperatures over a longer period while infusing it with the flavor of wood smoke.

- Use hardwood chunks, chips, or pellets to generate smoke. Common woods for smoking include hickory, mesquite, apple, and cherry.

2. Set Up Indirect Heat:

- On a charcoal grill, place the coals on one side and the food on the other for indirect heat. On a gas grill, use one burner for indirect cooking.

3. Water Pan:

- Place a water pan on the grill next to the coals. This helps maintain a moist cooking environment, which is essential for slow cooking.

4. Smoking Temperature:

- Maintain a low and consistent cooking temperature, typically between 225°F and 275°F (107°C to 135°C). Use a reliable thermometer to monitor the grill's temperature.

5. Patience:

- Smoking is a slow process. Be patient, and allow your food to smoke for the recommended time to develop that smoky flavor and tenderness.

III. Maintaining Heat in Outdoor Ovens

Outdoor ovens, such as wood-fired pizza ovens or brick ovens, provide an excellent platform for a wide range of cooking techniques, including baking pizzas, bread, and roasting meats. Here's how to maintain heat in outdoor ovens:

1. Heating the Oven:

- Start by building a fire inside the oven using wood or other suitable fuel. The type of wood you use can affect the flavor of your food.

2. Monitoring Temperature:

- Use a thermometer to monitor the oven's temperature. Wood-fired ovens can reach temperatures well above 700°F (370°C) for pizza, and lower temperatures (around 350-450°F or 175-230°C) for roasting.

3. Fire Management:

- Maintain a consistent fire by adding wood as needed. You can control the oven's temperature by adjusting the size and intensity of the fire.

4. Cooking Techniques:

- Wood-fired ovens are versatile and can be used for various techniques, including roasting, baking, and even smoking. The high heat produces a beautiful crust and smoky flavor.

5. Timing and Rotation:

- Pay attention to cooking times and rotate your food to ensure even cooking, especially in ovens with hot spots.

6. Use a Pizza Peel:

- A pizza peel is a handy tool for placing and retrieving food from the oven. It's especially useful for pizzas and bread.

IV. Safety Considerations

Outdoor cooking comes with some safety considerations:

1. Fire Safety:

- Always have a fire extinguisher nearby when using open flames. Keep a safe distance from flammable materials.

2. Food Safety:

- Practice safe food handling to prevent foodborne illnesses. Use a food thermometer to ensure that your food reaches safe internal temperatures.

3. Equipment Safety:

- Follow the manufacturer's instructions for your grill or outdoor oven. Regularly inspect and maintain your equipment for safety.

4. Ventilation:

- Ensure that your grilling area is well-ventilated to prevent the buildup of smoke and fumes.

5. Protective Gear:

- When working with high-temperature grills or ovens, use protective gear like oven mitts and long-handled tools to avoid burns.

Mastering the art of grilling and outdoor cooking is a rewarding journey that allows you to explore flavors, experiment with different techniques, and create memorable meals. With the right techniques and safety measures in place, you'll be well-equipped to take your outdoor culinary adventures to new heights, impressing family and friends with your delicious creations.

Chapter Fifteen

Specialty Appliances

Sous Vide Cooking, Griddles, Woks, and Specialty Pans, Toaster Ovens and Microwave Tips

Specialty appliances can elevate your cooking game, providing precision, versatility, and convenience in the kitchen. In this comprehensive guide, we'll explore the art of sous vide cooking, the benefits of griddles, woks, and specialty pans, and offer tips for getting the most out of your toaster oven and microwave. With these insights and techniques, you'll have a range of culinary tools at your disposal to create restaurant-quality dishes and streamline your cooking process.

I. Sous Vide Cooking: Precision at Its Best

Sous vide cooking is a culinary technique that involves cooking food in a precisely controlled water bath at a consistent low temperature. Here's how to master this method:

1. Equipment Needed:

- To get started with sous vide, you'll need an immersion circulator, a vacuum sealer (or resealable bags), and a container for the water bath.

2. Precise Temperature Control:

- Sous vide allows you to cook food to the exact desired done-ness. Use a digital thermometer to ensure the water bath's accuracy.

3. Vacuum Sealing:

- Vacuum-seal your ingredients to eliminate air and ensure even cooking. If you don't have a vacuum sealer, use the water displacement method with resealable bags.

4. Cooking Times:

- Consult sous vide cooking charts and guides for recommended times and temperatures for different foods. Cooking times can vary depending on the thickness of the food.

5. Searing:

- After sous vide cooking, give your food a quick sear in a hot pan or with a culinary torch to add flavor and texture.

II. Griddles, Woks, and Specialty Pans

Specialty pans offer unique cooking experiences and are essential for specific culinary styles. Here's how to make the most of griddles, woks, and specialty pans:

1. Griddles:

- Griddles are versatile for cooking pancakes, eggs, grilled cheese, and more. Preheat the griddle evenly and maintain a consistent temperature for even cooking.

2. Woks:

- A wok's high sides and sloping shape make it ideal for

stir-frying. Heat the wok until it's smoking hot, and have all your ingredients ready to cook quickly.

3. Specialty Pans:

- Specialty pans, like crepe pans or paella pans, are designed for specific dishes. Follow recipes and techniques tailored to these pans for best results.

III. Toaster Ovens and Microwave Tips

Toaster ovens and microwaves are convenient appliances for re-heating and cooking. Here are tips to maximize their use:

1. Toaster Ovens:

- Preheat your toaster oven for baking or roasting to ensure even cooking.

- Use the broil function to quickly brown the tops of dishes like casseroles or melt cheese.

2. Microwave Tips:

- Use microwave-safe containers and covers to prevent food splatters.

- When reheating, arrange food evenly in the dish for uniform heating.

- Stir or rotate food during microwave cooking to promote even cooking.

IV. Safety Considerations

Safety is paramount when using specialty appliances:

1. Sous Vide Safety:

- Ensure that the water bath's temperature remains constant to prevent foodborne illnesses.

- Use food-safe bags and materials for vacuum sealing.

2. Griddle and Wok Safety:

- Be cautious when working with hot griddles and woks. Use oven mitts or long-handled utensils to avoid burns.

3. Toaster Oven and Microwave Safety:

- Follow manufacturer guidelines for safe use of toaster ovens and microwaves.

- Avoid using metal cookware in microwaves to prevent sparking.

V. Cleaning and Maintenance

Proper cleaning and maintenance of specialty appliances ensure their longevity and safe use:

1. Sous Vide Circulator:

- Clean the immersion circulator after each use, and descale it periodically as recommended by the manufacturer.

2. Griddles and Pans:

- Clean specialty pans according to their materials (e.g., cast iron, non-stick). Avoid using abrasive scrubbers that can damage the surface.

3. Toaster Ovens and Microwaves:

- Regularly clean the interior and removable parts of these appliances to prevent buildup of food residues.

4. Safety Checks:

- Periodically inspect specialty appliances for any signs of wear, damage, or malfunction. Address any issues promptly.

By mastering these specialty appliances and techniques, you'll expand your culinary repertoire and create dishes with precision and convenience. Sous vide cooking will allow you to achieve perfect doneness every time, griddles and woks will add versatility to your cooking, and toaster ovens and microwaves will simplify your meal preparation. Remember to prioritize safety and proper maintenance to enjoy these appliances to the fullest.

Common Cooking Challenges

Overcooking and Undercooking, Hot Spots and Cold Spots, Rescuing Dishes Gone Awry

Cooking can be a delightful and rewarding experience, but it also comes with its fair share of challenges. Overcooking and undercooking, dealing with hot spots and cold spots, and rescuing dishes gone awry are all common issues in the kitchen. In this comprehensive guide, we'll address these cooking challenges and provide you with valuable tips and techniques to overcome them, ensuring your dishes turn out perfectly every time.

I. Overcooking and Undercooking: How to Avoid Them

One of the most common cooking challenges is achieving the right level of doneness. Overcooking and undercooking can result in less-than-perfect dishes. Here's how to avoid these pitfalls:

1. Use a Meat Thermometer:

- Invest in a reliable meat thermometer to accurately measure the internal temperature of meats. This ensures they reach the desired level of doneness without overcooking.

2. Rest Your Meat:

- After cooking meat, allow it to rest before slicing. This redistributes juices and ensures a tender, evenly cooked result.

3. Monitor Baking Times:

- For baked goods, set a timer and regularly check for doneness by inserting a toothpick or knife. If it comes out clean, your baked goods are ready.

4. Practice Stovetop Control:

- Adjust the heat on your stovetop as needed to prevent overcooking or undercooking. Cooking at the right temperature is key.

5. Follow Recipes Carefully:

- Pay attention to cooking times and temperatures specified in recipes. Slight variations can lead to overcooking or undercooking.

II. Hot Spots and Cold Spots: Troubleshooting Uneven Heat

Uneven heat distribution in ovens and stovetops can lead to uneven cooking. Here's how to troubleshoot and address hot spots and cold spots:

1. Oven Hot Spots:

- If your oven has hot spots, rotate dishes during baking to ensure even cooking.

- Consider using baking stones or pizza stones to help distribute heat more evenly.

2. Oven Cold Spots:

- Cold spots can result from poor insulation or faulty heating elements. If possible, have your oven serviced by a professional.

- Use an oven thermometer to identify and compensate for cold spots by adjusting cooking times and temperatures.

3. Stovetop Hot Spots:

- On stovetops with hot spots, move pans around to distribute heat more evenly.

- Use heavy-bottomed cookware, which can help mitigate hot spots.

4. Stovetop Cold Spots:

- If your stovetop has cold spots, be aware of their locations and adjust your cooking accordingly.

- Consider using cast iron pans, which retain and distribute heat more evenly.

III. Rescuing Dishes Gone Awry

Despite your best efforts, sometimes dishes don't turn out as planned. Here are some strategies for rescuing dishes that have gone awry:

1. Overcooked Meat:

- If meat is overcooked, try slicing it thinly and serving it with a flavorful sauce or gravy to add moisture and flavor.

2. Overcooked Vegetables:

- Overcooked vegetables can be pureed and turned into soups, sauces, or dips.

3. Salvaging Dry Baked Goods:

- For dry cakes or bread, brush them with a simple syrup or sugar glaze to add moisture.

4. Too Much Salt:

- If a dish is too salty, try adding unsalted ingredients to balance the flavors, such as extra vegetables, grains, or dairy.

5. Adjust Seasoning:

- Taste your dish and adjust seasoning as needed. Sometimes, a pinch of sugar or acid (like lemon juice or vinegar) can balance excessive saltiness.

6. Fix Overly Spicy Dishes:

- To mellow the heat in an overly spicy dish, add dairy products like yogurt, sour cream, or coconut milk.

7. Rescue Burnt Rice:

- If the bottom layer of rice is burnt, transfer the unburnt portion to a clean pot, add a bit of water, and steam it to soften and refresh the rice.

IV. Kitchen Tools to Help:

1. Heat Diffusers:

- Heat diffusers can be placed between your cookware and the heat source to help distribute heat evenly.

2. Oven Thermometer:

- An oven thermometer can accurately measure your oven's temperature and help identify hot spots or cold spots.

3. Quality Cookware:

- Invest in high-quality, heavy-bottomed cookware to promote even heat distribution.

4. Resting Rack:

- A resting rack or cutting board allows meat to rest without sitting in its juices, ensuring a crispy crust and juicy interior.

V. Safety and Maintenance:

1. Safety First:

- When troubleshooting cooking challenges, prioritize safety. Use oven mitts, pot holders, and utensils to protect yourself from hot cookware and surfaces.

2. Appliance Maintenance:

- Regularly clean and maintain your cooking appliances to ensure they function optimally. Check for any signs of damage or malfunction.

3. Practice Patience:

- Cooking can sometimes be a test of patience. Experimenting, learning from mistakes, and practicing are essential for improving your cooking skills.

4. Ask for Help:

- Don't hesitate to seek advice from experienced cooks, chefs, or online cooking communities when faced with challenging cooking issues.

By understanding how to avoid overcooking and undercooking, troubleshoot hot spots and cold spots, and rescue dishes that haven't turned out as planned, you'll become a more confident and skillful cook. Cooking challenges are opportunities for growth, creativity, and the development of your culinary expertise. With practice and patience, you'll master the art of cooking and create delicious dishes every time.

Chapter Seventeen

Perfecting Your Timing

Timing and Temperature, Using Thermometers and Timers Effectively, Timing Tips for Multi-Dish Meals

Timing is a crucial aspect of cooking that can make the difference between a perfectly cooked meal and one that falls short. In this comprehensive guide, we'll explore the art of perfect timing in the kitchen, including the relationship between timing and temperature, using thermometers and timers effectively, and providing timing tips for preparing multi-dish meals. With these insights and techniques, you'll be well-equipped to ensure that all components of your meal are ready to be served at their peak.

I. Timing and Temperature: The Perfect Duo

Timing and temperature go hand in hand in the culinary world. Understanding this dynamic is essential for achieving perfectly cooked dishes:

1. Temperature Control:

- Maintain control over cooking temperatures by using stovetops, ovens, grills, and other appliances effectively. Adjust heat levels as needed to avoid overcooking or undercooking.

2. Timing Precision:

- Timing is critical, especially when preparing dishes that require precise cooking times. Use timers to track cooking intervals accurately.

3. Food Thermometers:

- Invest in reliable food thermometers to measure the internal temperature of meats, poultry, and other foods. This ensures they reach the desired level of doneness.

4. Resting Time:

- Understand the importance of resting time for meats and certain dishes. Allow food to rest after cooking to redistribute juices and enhance flavor.

II. Using Thermometers and Timers Effectively

To perfect your timing in cooking, it's crucial to use thermometers and timers effectively:

1. Digital Meat Thermometers:

- Use digital meat thermometers with easy-to-read displays. Insert the probe into the thickest part of the meat without touching bone for accurate readings.

2. Instant-Read Thermometers:

- Instant-read thermometers provide quick and accurate temperature readings. Use them to check the doneness of meats and other dishes without keeping the oven or grill open for too long.

3. Leave-In Thermometers:

- Leave-in thermometers are ideal for slow-cooked dishes. They allow you to monitor food temperature without repeatedly opening the oven or smoker.

4. Multiple Thermometers:

- For multi-dish meals, consider using multiple thermometers to track the doneness of different items simultaneously.

5. Set Timers:

- Use kitchen timers or smartphone timers to keep track of cooking intervals. Set timers for each dish to ensure nothing is overlooked.

6. Cross-Check Doneness:

- Cross-check doneness by using both a timer and a thermometer. Follow recommended cooking times and verify with temperature readings.

III. Timing Tips for Multi-Dish Meals

Preparing multiple dishes for a meal can be a juggling act. Here are some timing tips for coordinating the cooking of multiple dishes:

1. Plan Ahead:

- Create a detailed cooking schedule that includes start and finish times for each dish. Factor in resting times as well.

2. Sequence Matters:

- Consider the cooking times of each dish and their temperature requirements. Start with items that require the longest cooking times and gradually add faster-cooking dishes.

3. Prep in Advance:

- Prepare ingredients and do as much prep work as possible before you start cooking. This reduces last-minute stress and helps maintain control over timing.

4. Keep Warm:

- Use a warm oven or warming drawer to keep dishes at the right temperature while you finish other components of the meal.

5. Resting Time:

- Allow some flexibility in your meal schedule to accommodate resting times for meats and certain dishes.

6. Assign Roles:

- If you have help in the kitchen, assign roles to different cooks to manage various components of the meal.

7. Practice:

- Perfecting the timing of multi-dish meals takes practice. Don't be discouraged by initial challenges; with experience, you'll become more adept at coordination.

IV. Safety Considerations:

1. Food Safety:

- When using thermometers, ensure they are clean and sanitized to prevent cross-contamination.

- Follow recommended safe minimum internal temperatures for meats and poultry to avoid foodborne illnesses.

2. Appliance Safety:

- Practice safe use of cooking appliances and equipment to prevent accidents and injuries.

Perfecting your timing in the kitchen is an art that requires practice and attention to detail. By understanding the relationship between timing and temperature, using thermometers and timers effectively, and implementing timing strategies for multi-dish meals, you'll be able to consistently serve perfectly cooked and well-coordinated dishes that delight your family and guests.

Chapter Eighteen

Recipes for Even Heat

Breakfast Classics, Appetizers and Snacks, Main Courses and Side Dishes, Desserts and Baked Goods

Achieving even heat is essential for cooking success, and it's equally crucial when preparing a wide range of dishes. In this collection of recipes, we'll explore breakfast classics, appetizers and snacks, main courses and side dishes, and delightful desserts and baked goods. Each recipe is designed to help you master even heat in various culinary scenarios, ensuring your dishes turn out perfectly.

I. Breakfast Classics: Perfectly Cooked Start to the Day

1. Classic Fluffy Pancakes

- Achieving even heat on your griddle or pan is crucial for making pancakes that are evenly golden brown. Preheat your cooking surface, and use a ladle to pour consistent portions of batter. Flip them when bubbles form and pop on the surface.

2. Perfectly Poached Eggs

- Poaching eggs requires precise temperature control. Bring water to a gentle simmer (not a rolling boil), add a splash of vinegar, and carefully slide in the eggs. The whites should set while the yolks remain runny.

II. Appetizers and Snacks: Even Heat for Flavorful Bites

3. Crispy Potato Latkes

- Even heat is crucial for crispy latkes. Heat the oil in a skillet until it shimmers but doesn't smoke. Use a spoon to form evenly sized latkes, and fry until they're golden brown on both sides.

4. Baked Buffalo Chicken Wings

- Achieving even heat in the oven ensures crispy, evenly cooked chicken wings. Use a wire rack on a baking sheet to allow air circulation, and flip the wings halfway through the baking time for even crispness.

III. Main Courses and Side Dishes: Perfectly Balanced Flavors

5. Pan-Seared Steak

- Even heat is essential for achieving a perfect sear on a steak. Preheat your skillet or pan until it's smoking hot. Sear the steak for a few minutes on each side to develop a beautiful crust while keeping the inside juicy.

6. Risotto with Mushrooms

- Risotto relies on even heat for a creamy texture. Use a heavy-bottomed pan, add warm broth gradually, and stir constantly. The rice should cook evenly and absorb the liquid without sticking.

IV. Desserts and Baked Goods: Sweet Perfection

7. Flourless Chocolate Cake

- Achieving even heat when baking a flourless chocolate cake is crucial to avoid overcooking the edges while keeping the center rich and fudgy. Use a water bath (bain-marie) for gentle and even baking.

8. Perfectly Golden Croissants

- Even heat in the oven is vital for perfectly golden, flaky croissants. Preheat your oven, and bake the croissants on a parchment-lined baking sheet until they're evenly browned and puffed.

V. Tips for Even Heat in All Recipes:

- **Preheat:** Always preheat your cooking surface or oven to the specified temperature in the recipe. This ensures that your food cooks evenly from the start.

- **Use Quality Cookware:** High-quality pots and pans with even heat distribution can make a significant difference in cooking results.

- **Rotate and Monitor:** When baking or roasting, rotate dishes halfway through cooking to ensure even browning. Use timers and thermometers to monitor progress.

- **Rest Meat:** Allow cooked meats to rest before slicing. This helps redistribute juices for even moisture throughout.

VI. Safety Considerations:

- **Hot Surfaces:** Be cautious of hot cooking surfaces and ovens to prevent burns and injuries.

- **Food Safety:** Practice safe food handling and hygiene to avoid foodborne illnesses.

By mastering the art of even heat in cooking, you'll be able to prepare these delicious breakfast classics, appetizers and snacks, main courses and side dishes, and desserts and baked goods with confidence. Each recipe showcases the importance of precise temperature control and even heat distribution for exceptional culinary results. Enjoy your culinary journey!

Chapter Nineteen

Beyond the Kitchen

Applying Even Heat to DIY Projects, Tips for Even Heat in Home Brewing, Heat-Related Science Experiments

Even heat isn't just essential in the kitchen; it plays a crucial role in various DIY projects, home brewing, and exciting science experiments. In this guide, we'll explore how to apply even heat in non-culinary scenarios, offer tips for maintaining consistent temperatures in home brewing, and provide heat-related science experiments for curious minds.

I. Applying Even Heat to DIY Projects

Even heat is vital in many DIY projects, whether you're working with wood, metal, or other materials. Here's a project idea where even heat is key:

1. Woodworking: Creating a Wood Finish

- Applying a wood finish requires even heat to ensure the finish spreads smoothly and evenly across the wood surface. Use a heat gun set to a low and consistent temperature to warm the finish and the wood, making it easier to apply and achieve a flawless result.

II. Tips for Even Heat in Home Brewing

Home brewing is a craft that relies heavily on precise temperature control to achieve the desired flavors in beer. Here are some tips for maintaining even heat in home brewing:

2. Mash Temperature Control

- Maintain a consistent mash temperature when brewing beer. Use a well-insulated mash tun or vessel to prevent temperature fluctuations during the mashing process.

3. Boil Vigilance

- During the boiling stage, use a reliable heat source, such as a propane burner, with precise control. A rolling boil should be maintained consistently to extract the desired flavors and aromas.

4. Fermentation Temperature

- Keep a close eye on fermentation temperature, as it can greatly affect the final flavor of your beer. Use a fermentation chamber or temperature-controlled environment to ensure even and stable heat.

III. Heat-Related Science Experiments

Exploring heat through science experiments is not only educational but also a lot of fun. Here are some heat-related science experiments suitable for various age groups:

5. Solar Oven Experiment

- Build a simple solar oven using materials like cardboard, aluminum foil, and plastic wrap. Test its ability to harness the sun's heat to cook food or melt chocolate.

6. Water Temperature and Dissolving Rates

- Investigate how different water temperatures affect the rate at which substances like sugar or salt dissolve. Use a controlled heat source to vary the water's temperature.

7. Thermal Expansion with Balloons

- Observe the concept of thermal expansion by placing an inflated balloon over the neck of a bottle. Submerge the bottle in hot water, and watch as the balloon expands due to the heat.

8. Heat and Melting Points

- Explore the melting points of various substances, such as chocolate, crayons, or ice, using different heat sources like stovetops, ovens, or hot plates.

9. Insulating Materials

- Test different insulating materials, such as foam, cloth, or paper, to see which one best retains heat. Use a heat source like a light bulb or heat lamp to provide consistent warmth.

10. The Boiling Water Challenge

- Challenge participants to predict the time it takes for a given volume of water to reach a rolling boil under different heating conditions, such as using a stovetop, microwave, or kettle.

Safety Considerations for DIY Projects and Science Experiments:

- **Supervision:** Ensure proper supervision, especially when conducting heat-related experiments with children.

- **Safety Gear:** Use appropriate safety gear, such as goggles, gloves, and heat-resistant materials, when necessary.

- **Follow Instructions:** Always follow instructions and guidelines for the specific DIY project or science experiment to avoid accidents or injuries.

Exploring the applications of even heat beyond the kitchen opens up exciting opportunities for creativity, learning, and discovery. Whether you're working on DIY projects, home brewing, or engaging in heat-related science experiments, understanding the principles of even heat will help you achieve your goals effectively and safely. Enjoy your adventures beyond the kitchen!

Chapter Twenty

Recap of Key Takeaways

Embracing Even Heat in Your Culinary Journey

In the world of cooking, the pursuit of even heat is a fundamental principle that can make or break your culinary creations. Whether you're a novice cook or a seasoned chef, mastering the art of even heat is essential for consistently delicious and well-cooked dishes. In this comprehensive recap, we'll revisit the key takeaways on how to embrace even heat in your culinary journey.

I. The Significance of Even Heat

1. Temperature Consistency:

- Even heat ensures that all parts of your cooking surface or oven are at the same temperature, preventing uneven cooking or burning.

2. Precise Doneness:

- Achieving even heat allows you to cook ingredients to the desired level of doneness, whether it's a perfectly seared steak, a golden-brown pancake, or a tender roast.

3. Flavor Development:

- Even heat promotes uniform flavor development by allowing ingredients to cook evenly and absorb seasonings consistently.

II. The Science of Heat Transfer

4. Conduction:

- Conduction is the direct transfer of heat from one surface to another through direct contact, like when a pan heats up and cooks food touching its surface.

5. Convection:

- Convection involves the circulation of heat through a fluid, such as air or liquid. This method is used in ovens and stovetops to distribute heat evenly.

6. Radiation:

- Radiation is the transfer of heat through electromagnetic waves, as seen in grilling or broiling.

III. Achieving Even Heat in Cooking

7. Preheating:

- Always preheat your cooking surface or oven to the desired temperature before adding your ingredients. This ensures a consistent starting point.

8. Quality Cookware:

- Invest in high-quality pots, pans, and bakeware that distribute heat evenly.

9. Control Your Heat Source:

- Adjust the intensity of your heat source, whether it's a stove-top burner or an oven, to maintain even cooking.

10. Tools of Precision:

- Use tools like food thermometers and timers to monitor temperatures and cooking times accurately.

IV. Cooking Techniques for Even Heat

11. Searing:

- Achieve a perfect sear on meats by using a hot, even surface. Searing locks in juices and enhances flavor.

12. Baking and Roasting:

- Bake and roast with even heat for consistent browning and cooking throughout.

13. Sous Vide:

- Sous vide cooking relies on precise temperature control to cook food to perfection.

14. Resting Time:

- Allow cooked meats and dishes to rest before serving to redistribute juices for even moisture.

V. Troubleshooting Even Heat Challenges

15. Overcooking and Undercooking:

- Use meat thermometers and precise timing to avoid these common pitfalls.

16. Hot Spots and Cold Spots:

- Address uneven heat distribution by rotating dishes or using tools like baking stones.

17. Rescuing Dishes Gone Awry:

- Salvage overcooked or overly spicy dishes with creative fixes.

VI. Perfecting Your Timing

18. Timing and Temperature:

- Understand the relationship between timing and temperature for perfectly cooked dishes.

19. Using Thermometers and Timers Effectively:

- Use digital meat thermometers and timers to achieve precise cooking results.

20. Timing Tips for Multi-Dish Meals:

- Plan, sequence, and coordinate your cooking to ensure all components of a meal are ready simultaneously.

VII. Recipes for Even Heat

21. Breakfast Classics:

- Master the art of evenly cooking pancakes and poaching eggs for a delicious start to your day.

22. Appetizers and Snacks:

- Achieve even heat for crispy potato latkes and perfectly baked buffalo chicken wings.

23. Main Courses and Side Dishes:

- Create evenly seared steaks and creamy mushroom risotto for satisfying meals.

24. Desserts and Baked Goods:

- Achieve even heat when baking flourless chocolate cake and golden croissants for sweet perfection.

VIII. Beyond the Kitchen

25. Applying Even Heat to DIY Projects:

- Apply even heat to DIY projects, such as achieving a smooth wood finish with a heat gun.

26. Tips for Even Heat in Home Brewing:

- Maintain even temperatures during home brewing to create consistent and flavorful beer.

27. Heat-Related Science Experiments:

- Explore heat-related science experiments, from solar ovens to thermal expansion demonstrations.

IX. Conclusion

Embracing even heat in your culinary journey is a journey in itself, one that involves science, precision, and creativity. With a deep understanding of the principles of even heat, you can confidently tackle a wide range of dishes, troubleshoot cooking challenges, perfect your timing, and even apply these principles beyond the kitchen. As you continue to hone your culinary skills, remember that even heat is your ally, guiding you toward culinary excellence and delicious meals that will delight your family and guests. Happy cooking!

Temperature Conversion Charts

Fahrenheit to Celsius and Celsius to Fahrenheit

Temperature conversions are essential for understanding temperature scales commonly used in different parts of the world. Here are charts to help you easily convert temperatures between Fahrenheit and Celsius:

Fahrenheit to Celsius Conversion Chart:

- -50°F = -45.56°C

- -40°F = -40.00°C

- -30°F = -34.44°C

- -20°F = -28.89°C

- -10°F = -23.33°C

- 0°F = -17.78°C

- 10°F = -12.22°C

- 20°F = -6.67°C

- 30°F = -1.11°C

- 40°F = 4.44°C

- 50°F = 10.00°C

- 60°F = 15.56°C

- 70°F = 21.11°C

- 80°F = 26.67°C

- 90°F = 32.22°C

- 100°F = 37.78°C

- 110°F = 43.33°C

- 120°F = 48.89°C

- 130°F = 54.44°C

- 140°F = 60.00°C

- 150°F = 65.56°C

- 160°F = 71.11°C

- **170°F = 76.67°C**

- **180°F = 82.22°C**

- **190°F = 87.78°C**

- **200°F = 93.33°C**

- **212°F (Boiling Point of Water) = 100.00°C**

Celsius to Fahrenheit Conversion Chart:

- **-50°C = -58°F**

- **-40°C = -40°F**

- **-30°C = -22°F**

- **-20°C = -4°F**

- **-10°C = 14°F**

- **0°C = 32°F**

- **10°C = 50°F**

- **20°C = 68°F**

- **30°C = 86°F**

- **40°C = 104°F**

- **50°C = 122°F**

- **60°C = 140°F**

- **70°C = 158°F**

- **80°C = 176°F**

- **90°C = 194°F**

- **100°C = 212°F**

- **110°C = 230°F**

- **120°C = 248°F**

- **130°C = 266°F**

- **140°C = 284°F**

- **150°C = 302°F**

- **160°C = 320°F**

- **170°C = 338°F**

- **180°C = 356°F**

- **190°C = 374°F**

- **200°C = 392°F**

These conversion charts will assist you in converting temperatures accurately between Fahrenheit and Celsius, whether you're working with recipes, weather forecasts, or any situation where temperature units differ.

Chapter Twenty-Two

Cooking Equipment Guide

Recommended Cookware and Utensils

When it comes to equipping your kitchen for culinary adventures, having the right cookware and utensils can make a world of difference. Whether you're a novice cook or an experienced chef, the quality and variety of your tools play a crucial role in the success of your dishes. In this comprehensive guide, we'll explore recommended cookware and utensils for a well-equipped kitchen, along with some brands and models to consider.

I. Essential Cookware: The Foundation of Your Kitchen

1. **Skillets/Frying Pans:**

   - **Recommendation:** All-Clad Stainless Steel Fry Pan, Lodge Cast Iron Skillet

   - Skillets are versatile and essential for searing, frying, sautéing, and more. Stainless steel and cast iron options are highly durable.

2. **Saucepans:**

- **Recommendation:** Cuisinart MultiClad Pro Saucepan, Le Creuset Enameled Cast Iron Saucepan

- Saucepans are used for simmering, boiling, and making sauces. Look for a variety of sizes to accommodate different cooking needs.

3. **Stockpot:**

- **Recommendation:** All-Clad Stainless Steel Stockpot, Calphalon Contemporary Nonstick Stockpot

- A stockpot is perfect for making soups, stews, stocks, and pasta. Consider one with a sturdy handle and a lid.

4. **Dutch Oven:**

- **Recommendation:** Lodge Cast Iron Dutch Oven, Le Creuset Enameled Cast Iron Dutch Oven

- Dutch ovens are great for slow cooking, roasting, braising, and baking. Enameled cast iron options offer even heat distribution.

5. **Baking Sheets:**

- **Recommendation:** Nordic Ware Natural Aluminum Commercial Baker's Half Sheet, USA Pan Bakeware Half Sheet Pan

- Baking sheets are essential for roasting vegetables, baking cookies, and more. Opt for heavy-duty, nonstick models.

6. Casserole Dish:

- **Recommendation:** Pyrex Easy Grab Glass Casserole Dish, Le Creuset Stoneware Casserole Dish

- Casserole dishes are perfect for oven-baked dishes like lasagna, casseroles, and gratins. Choose one that's oven-safe and stylish.

II. Specialized Cookware: Enhancing Your Culinary Repertoire

1. Nonstick Skillet:

- **Recommendation:** T-fal E76507 Ultimate Hard Anodized Nonstick Fry Pan, Calphalon Contemporary Nonstick Omelette Fry Pan

- Nonstick skillets are great for cooking eggs, delicate foods, and dishes that require minimal oil.

2. Grill Pan:

- **Recommendation:** Lodge Pro-Grid Cast Iron Grill and Griddle Combo, Calphalon Contemporary Nonstick Square Grill Pan

- Grill pans are ideal for achieving grill marks and flavors indoors, especially for meats and vegetables.

3. Wok:

- **Recommendation:** Joyce Chen Pro Chef Flat Bottom Wok, Lodge Pro-Logic Cast Iron Wok

- A wok is essential for stir-frying, and a flat bottom design is suitable for various stovetops.

4. **Roasting Pan:**

- **Recommendation:** Cuisinart Chef's Classic Stainless Steel Roaster, Viking 3-Ply Stainless Steel Roasting Pan

- Roasting pans are necessary for cooking large cuts of meat, poultry, and roasts. Look for models with a rack.

III. Essential Utensils: Tools of Precision and Control
1. Chef's Knife:

- **Recommendation:** Wusthof Classic Chef's Knife, Victorinox Fibrox Pro Chef's Knife

- A high-quality chef's knife is indispensable for slicing, dicing, and chopping. Choose one that feels comfortable in your hand.

2. Paring Knife:

- **Recommendation:** Mercer Culinary Genesis Forged Paring Knife, Zwilling J.A. Henckels Pro Paring Knife

- Paring knives are ideal for intricate tasks like peeling and trimming fruits and vegetables.

3. Cutting Board:

- **Recommendation:** OXO Good Grips Utility Cutting Board, John Boos Maple Wood Reversible Cutting Board

- Durable cutting boards protect your knives and provide ample space for slicing and chopping.

4. **Tongs:**

- **Recommendation:** OXO Good Grips 12-Inch Stainless-Steel Locking Tongs, Winco Utility Tong

- Tongs are versatile for flipping, tossing, and serving a wide range of dishes.

5. **Whisk:**

- **Recommendation:** Winco Stainless Steel French Whip, OXO Good Grips Better Flat Wire Whisk

- Whisks are essential for blending, emulsifying, and whipping ingredients smoothly.

IV. Brands and Models to Consider:

- **All-Clad:** Known for high-quality stainless steel cookware.

- **Le Creuset:** Renowned for colorful enameled cast iron pieces.

- **Lodge:** Trusted for affordable and durable cast iron cookware.

- **Calphalon:** Offers a wide range of nonstick and stainless steel options.

- **Cuisinart:** Known for versatile and affordable kitchen appliances.

- **T-fal:** Recognized for its nonstick cookware and innovative designs.

- **Wusthof:** A top choice for precision knives and cutlery.

- **OXO:** Known for ergonomic and user-friendly kitchen tools.

- **John Boos:** Renowned for high-quality wooden cutting boards.

Having the right cookware and utensils enhances your cooking experience and allows you to tackle a variety of recipes with confidence. When choosing kitchen equipment, consider your cooking style, budget, and the specific needs of your kitchen. With the right tools at your disposal, you can unleash your culinary creativity and create delicious meals for yourself and your loved ones.

Chapter Twenty-Three

References

1. "The Joy of Cooking" by Irma S. Rombauer and Marion Rombauer Becker

2. "Essentials of Classic Italian Cooking" by Marcella Hazan

3. "Salt, Fat, Acid, Heat" by Samin Nosrat

4. "The Food Lab: Better Home Cooking Through Science" by J. Kenji López-Alt

5. "Vegetable Kingdom: The Abundant World of Vegan Recipes" by Bryant Terry

Chapter Twenty-Four

Glossary

Key Terms and Concepts in Cooking and Culinary Arts

Cooking and culinary arts encompass a rich vocabulary of terms and concepts. Understanding these key terms is essential for becoming a proficient cook. Here's a glossary to help you navigate the world of cooking:

1. Blanching:

- A cooking technique where food is briefly boiled, then immediately plunged into ice water to stop the cooking process. It's often used for vegetables to retain their color and texture.

2. Braising:

- A method of cooking that involves searing meat or vegetables in fat, then slowly simmering them in a flavorful liquid, often covered. This results in tender and well-flavored dishes.

3. Deglaze:

- To add liquid (usually wine or broth) to a hot pan to dissolve and release browned bits of food that have stuck to the bottom. This process enhances sauces and gravies.

4. Emulsify:

- To mix two immiscible liquids, such as oil and vinegar, into a stable and uniform mixture, typically using an emulsifying agent like egg yolk or mustard.

5. Julienne:

- To cut food, usually vegetables, into thin, matchstick-sized strips.

6. Mirepoix:

- A classic flavor base in French cuisine made from diced onions, carrots, and celery. It's used to add depth and aroma to soups, sauces, and stews.

7. Poach:

- To gently cook food, often delicate items like eggs or fish, by submerging them in simmering liquid until they're just cooked.

8. Roux:

- A mixture of fat (usually butter) and flour used as a thickening agent for sauces, gravies, and soups.

9. Sauté:

- A quick cooking method that involves cooking small pieces of food in a small amount of oil or butter over high heat. It's used for browning and developing flavor.

10. Sear:

- To brown the surface of meat, poultry, or fish quickly over high heat to lock in juices and add flavor.

11. Sous Vide:

- A cooking method where food is vacuum-sealed in a bag and cooked in a precisely controlled water bath at a specific temperature, resulting in evenly cooked and tender dishes.

12. Tofu:

- A protein-rich food made from soybean curds. It's a versatile ingredient in vegetarian and vegan cooking.

13. Zest:

- The outer, colored part of citrus fruit peel, typically grated or thinly sliced and used to add flavor to dishes.

14. Al Dente:

- An Italian term meaning "to the tooth." It describes pasta or other grains that are cooked until they are still slightly firm when bitten.

15. Bain-Marie:

- A water bath used to gently and evenly heat delicate dishes like custards and sauces. It provides a gentle and indirect source of heat.

16. Caramelization:

- The process of browning sugars in food through the application of heat. It results in a complex, sweet flavor and a characteristic brown color.

17. Mise en Place:

- A French term that means "everything in its place." It refers to the practice of prepping and organizing all ingredients before starting cooking to ensure a smooth cooking process.

18. Reduction:

- The process of simmering a liquid, such as a sauce or stock, to evaporate water and concentrate flavors, resulting in a thicker consistency.

19. Umami:

- One of the five basic tastes, characterized as savory and often described as a rich and meaty flavor. Umami is found in foods like tomatoes, mushrooms, and soy sauce.

20. Blanch:

- To briefly cook food in boiling water, then immediately cool it in ice water. It's used for various purposes, including peeling fruits or vegetables and preserving color and texture.

This glossary provides a foundation for understanding essential cooking terms and concepts. As you explore the culinary world, you'll encounter many more specialized terms and techniques that will enhance your cooking skills and repertoire.

9 798864 498491